TEN
SPICES
FOR
HEALTH
AND
LONGEVITY

By

Valerie B. Lull

Other Books by Valerie Lull

Ten Healthy Teas

Table of Contents

1) Cinnamon....................8

2) Ginger....................15

3) Cayenne....................21

4) Sage....................26

5) Rosemary....................31

6) Thyme....................38

7) Basil....................45

8) Oregano....................51

9) Turmeric....................56

10) Clove....................61

Dedication

To Maija, Louise, Susan and Shirley

Why I Have Written this Book

I have always been interested in health and things that help people stay healthy. At the age of 58, I made a career change from mental health and studied to be a Master Herbalist. I learned many new things that are really quite simple and easy to do that would help folks stay healthy. I decided I wanted to share this information with people, especially people that are interested in healthful things but may not know a whole lot about it. Many of these folks would like to know more but don't know where to start.

My book is meant to be a guide to show how really easy it is to do simple things that extend life and promote health. I started out with my first book, *Ten Healthy Teas,* and now I am delving into the world of healthful spices.

Many of the spices we are familiar with have healing properties as well as culinary uses and are very inexpensive to buy. Many spices are as close as the produce department in your local market. Spices are used in everyday cooking, as teas, as supplements and essential oils.

In writing this book I found it hard to narrow it down to 10 spices. There are so many good spices that have good health qualities. There are many plants that are considered to be both herbs and spices, for example, cinnamon. It is a popular spice used often in desserts, but it is also considered to be an herb and has medicinal uses. Most people put spices in the culinary category and don't think about their healing properties, but spices have health benefits as well. Many of them can be made into teas that are therapeutic.

Healthy spices can also come in the form of essential oils. These are used a lot in aromatherapy, and massage therapy. Most essential oils cannot be taken orally. Be careful; some can be poisonous. Be sure you know what you are doing if you want to take essential oils orally. Always check with your health care provider before starting to use essential oils, herbs or supplements.

I hope you will join me on this journey into the world of spices and vibrant health.

--Valerie Lull

Disclaimer

The information contained in this book is not intended to replace professional medical advice. Any use of the information in this book is at the reader's discretion. The author and publisher specifically disclaim any and all liability arising directly or indirectly from the use or application of any information contained in this book. A health care professional should always be consulted about your specific situation.

1) Cinnamon

Cinnamon is one spice that I really like. It is like an accent to a good food, like sprinkling cinnamon on applesauce, or your morning oatmeal. It tastes good and it is good for you.

There are two kinds of cinnamon, *cinnamomum cassia*, also called Chinese cinnamon, and *Cinnamomum zeylanicum* known as Ceylon cinnamon. Cassia is from China and is the kind that is used the most in the United States. It is sweeter and stronger than the Ceylon kind.

Cinnamon is called by some people a winter spice. This is probably because it is used in so many of the foods prepared during the holiday season. Who can resist cinnamon buns, or baked apples with cinnamon, walnuts and raisins in them or putting a cinnamon stick in a cup of hot tea or coco.

Cinnamon is one of a number of spices that are both an herb and a spice. It is good for both culinary and therapeutic purposes. There's some promising research on the use of cinnamon for controlling blood sugar. Recent findings seem to support the use of cinnamon for diabetes. It said to bring down blood sugar. It is also said to support uses for flatulence, muscle spasms, preventing vomiting, diarrhea, infections, common cold, the loss of appetite, impotence, lowering cholesterol, and menopausal symptoms.

Some of the additional properties of garlic are that it is anti-inflammatory, anti-bacterial, ant repellent, and anti-fungal. But, don't go to the spice section in the supermarket and start downing bottles of cinnamon. You could get too much.

Cinnamon was used by the ancients. The Romans, who believed cinnamon was sacred, burned it at funerals. History tells us that Nero burned cinnamon at his wife's funeral. Cinnamon is also an important herb in the Traditional Chinese Medicine compilation called *Materia Medica*.

In Chinese medicine cinnamon was used to treat a wide variety of disorders characterized by intolerance to cold, cold limbs, weakness, soreness, coldness of the low back and knees, impotence, low libido, and loose bowel movements. Cinnamon was and still is used to treat digestive disorders that according to traditional Chinese medical philosophy are cold in nature. These may manifest as stomach pain and diarrhea. The volatile oils in cinnamon appear to have a mild stimulating action on digestion. They dispel gas, and relieve spasmodic pain in the stomach and intestines.

Also, in traditional Chinese medicine, the sliced twigs of the cinnamon tree are used, and are in the category of warming diaphoretics, which is herbal language for an herb that makes you sweat. These twigs have also been used for pain and stiffness in the superficial layers of the body such as muscles and joints when the pain and stiffness are due to cold and damp. Cinnamon twigs can also be used as a guiding herb that leads other herbs to specific parts of the body.

There are other species of cinnamon such as *C. burmunii* that will warm the digestion, but they are not used therapeutically as they are mild in nature. They are used in cooking and baking. Cinnamon has many uses and is excellent both as food and medicine.

Cinnamon can flavor fruits, vegetables, rice, and hot coco. Cinnamon sticks go great in both herbal tisanes and teas. Cinnamon suppresses the growth of E. coli and other strains of bacteria. It may prevent or slow type II diabetes and help lower blood sugar.

Cinnamon is often used as part of a tea blend to improve the taste of other less tasty herbs. It has powerful antibacterial properties which can be added to cold and flu remedies. Cinnamon can also make a good tasting tea all by itself. Cinnamon is a good spice to keep on hand for whenever the occasion calls for it.

Side Effects:

Large amounts of cinnamon over a long period of time may cause some people to bleed excessively and Cassia oil can irritate the skin.

Cinnamon can also cause an increase in heart rate, inflammation in the mouth, difficulty breathing, upset stomach, loose stools, and allergic reactions. Essential oil of cinnamon that is applied to the skin may cause burning and irritation. Women who are pregnant or nursing should avoid using cinnamon in medicinal doses.

Cinnamon can thin the blood, so don't take it before surgery or if you are taking blood thinners. Cinnamon is often used for folks with diabetes because it makes the blood sugar go down, but don't try to use it without consulting your health care practitioner. Your blood sugar could go too low. Cinnamon may also interact with antibiotics. Again, consult your medical provider.

RECIPES

NOTE: Many spices are also herbs and can be used as teas. A tea is 1 teaspoon herb or spice, and 1 C boiling water. It steeps anywhere from 2 to 10 minutes depending on how strong you want it. Don't store the tea for more than 24 hours. An infusion is 1 oz. spice or herb and 1 pint water that will steep for 20 minutes. A decoction is usually used for roots, bark and stems and is made in a saucepan. Enamel or stainless steel works best. Never use aluminum. It is made with 1 oz. bark, root or stems, and 1 pint water. It simmers until ¼ of the water has gone down. Strain the decoction and use. Do not store in the refrigerator for more than 24 hours.

Cinnamon Tea

Many fine teas are made with blends of cinnamon and other spices and fruits and herbs. Cinnamon alone can make a fine tea. It can also be added to teas that do not taste good to improve the flavor. Here is the simple recipe:

1 stick of cinnamon, use a small stick and break it in half for 1-2 cups of boiling water.

Sweeten as desired. You can use honey, stevia, or your own favorite sweetener. Agave syrup and maple syrup are other good options.

Add boiling water and steep for 10 minutes. Using powdered cinnamon will make the tea cloudy.

Breakfast rice with cinnamon

1 bowl cooked rice, white or brown, either is ok

1 t cinnamon

1 t brown sugar

Butter, as much as desired and/or milk

Mix ingredients and enjoy.

Additional Uses:

Air freshener – Put a few drops of cinnamon essential oil on a cool light bulb so that it can diffuse throughout the room. Another way to freshen the air is to put some cinnamon in small dishes, and distribute them around your home. A third way to use cinnamon to freshen the air is to mix a few drops of cinnamon essential oil with water, put it in a spray bottle and spray it around the house. It helps to get rid of germs and unwanted odors.

Ant repellent – Sprinkle some cinnamon in the places where the ants come in and on their regular trails. You can also make a spray. Put cinnamon essential oil and vinegar in a spray bottle. Use about 100 drops of cinnamon essential oil and add one cup of vinegar. Spray where the ants come in and on their trails.

Incense – Cinnamon incense can be bought and you can burn it in your home, or you can put some cinnamon in a dish that is heat proof and light it and burn it.

Massage- Mix a few drops of cinnamon essential oil with a carrier oil and use it for massage. It is warming to the body.

Moth repellent – Mix some broken cinnamon sticks with cloves and black peppercorns. Put in little cloth sacks and hang in your closet or any other place where you want to get rid of moths.

2) Ginger

The spice known as ginger is the underground rhizome of the ginger plant, known botanically as *Zingiber officinale*. Ginger is another one of my favorite spices. I like to drink ginger tea on cool fall and winter mornings. It warms me up and helps my arthritis. Ginger has been used extensively in cakes, cookies and Asian cuisine. Besides its culinary uses ginger is also useful for healing purposes. It was a favorite spice for cooking and healing in ancient China and Rome. In Chinese medicine it is considered a warming herb.

In both Traditional Chinese medicine and in Ayeurveda (the medicine of India) ginger is mentioned in the earliest writings. It is used extensively in Traditional Chinese medicine for colds and for its usefulness in detoxifying the body and raising body heat. In Chinese medicine ginger is called Gan-jiang for dried ginger and Sheg-jiang for fresh ginger. Juice squeezed from the root is used for burns and ginger is used in at least half of all the Chinese medications. It is believed that ginger in moderation can strengthen the lungs and kidneys.

If you are traveling and have problems with motion sickness, ginger is a good remedy to have on hand. In addition to helping digestive problems ginger is an anti-inflammatory. Ginger is good for upset stomach, nausea, body aches, arthritis, and motion sickness. Some folks find it relaxing and calming.

In the past ginger has been used for morning sickness. In recent times pregnant women have been told not to use it because it stimulates the uterus. This remains a controversial issue and the current recommendation is not to use ginger any more than would be consumed as a spice for food. Always check with your health care provider before taking ginger, especially if you are pregnant.

In the world of herbs ginger has been used in herbal formulas to disguise the taste of other herbs that don't taste good. In some formulas it increases potency which means it helps in speeding up the action of the formula.

Ginger is said to be a blood thinner and may help angina pains. It increases blood flow, which helps relieve abdominal cramps and bring on menstruation. Ginger has been used for the relief of pain from arthritis, cough, bronchitis, chest pain, low back pain and stomach pain.

Ginger oil is used in massage blends. It has a spicy-woody odor. It warms the body and relaxes tight, sore muscles. It is useful for controlling nausea from chemotherapy. It improves digestion and can prevent indigestion. Ginger combines well in herbal formulas and with turmeric which is also anti-inflammatory and pain-relieving. Ginger is a carminative. That means it helps flatulence or intestinal gas. It causes the intestinal tract to relax and it is soothing.

According to modern research ginger possesses antioxidants and is anti-inflammatory. The anti-inflammatory effects of ginger are substances called gingerols. The gingerols help relieve pain from arthritis, both osteoarthritis and rheumatoid arthritis. Gingerols may inhibit the growth of colon cancer cells. Recent research also suggests that gingerols may also kill ovarian cancer cells. Ginger may also be anti-tumor.

Ginger may cause sweating, which is a good thing when folks have colds or flu. Sweating aids in detoxification of the body. Fresh ginger seems to be more potent then dried ginger.

Side Effects

Pregnant women are cautioned regarding the use of ginger because it is a uterine stimulant. If you are pregnant and want to use ginger discuss it with your health care provider. Side effects are not common.

Do not take ginger if you are on a blood-thinning medication, or an aspirin regimen. People with heart problems, gallstones and diabetes should ask their doctors before starting ginger. In high doses ginger may cause heartburn, diarrhea and irritation of the mouth. Some of this may be avoided if the ginger is taken with meals.

Ginger may interact with some medications like warfarin (Coumadin), or clopidogrel (Plavix). In people with diabetes it may also lower blood sugar. Ginger may interact with blood pressure medications. Be sure to consult your doctor before using ginger for medicinal purposes.

Do not give ginger to children under two. If you want to give it to older children, consult your health care professional for the right dosage.

RECIPES

NOTE: Ginger is another spice/tea that can be used to improve the flavor of teas that do not taste good.

Ginger Ale Punch

1 Qt. ginger ale

1 Qt. apple or cranberry juice or cranapple juice

A pinch of cinnamon

Mix ingredients. Chill and/or add ice. Serve and enjoy!

Fresh Ginger Tea

4-6 thin slices raw ginger, more for a stronger tea

1 1/2 - 2 C water

Juice from ½ lemon

1-2 T honey or sweetener of choice

Preparation:

Peel the ginger and slice thinly.

Boil the ginger in water for at least 10 minutes. For a stronger tea, allow to boil for 20 minutes or more, and use more slices of ginger.

Remove from heat and add lemon and honey or sweetener of choice. Enjoy!

Ginger and Honey (for digestion)

One piece of fresh ginger 3-4 inches long

1 teaspoon honey

Water

Peel ginger. Put it in a blender with water to crush it. Remove from blender and squeeze out the juice. Filter the juice. Add honey. Mix well and drink.

This recipe is good for food poisoning as well as for an upset stomach.

Additional Uses:

Anti-inflammatory – Ginger extract has anti-inflammatory properties.

Bath - If you have sore muscles, arthritis, or fibromyalgia, you can take a soothing and detoxifying bath with rosemary and ginger combined.

Circulation – Ginger added to food aids the blood circulation.

Lemonade – Add ginger to your lemonade for an additional zing.

Lung congestion – A ginger poultice is good for lung congestion

Massage – Ginger can be blended with other oils to relieve sore muscles and cause relaxation.

3) Cayenne

Cayenne, known in Latin as *Capsicum annuum,* is a member of the *capsicium* family. Cayenne is an interesting spice. It is part of the family of peppers, like jalapeno, habanero, chili peppers, bell peppers and more. It is known for its spicy heat and if you eat enough, it will make you sweat. This makes it great for sweating toxins out of your body.

Cayenne peppers and other peppers in the same family are native to South and Central America. These cultures are famous for their spicy hot food. The early explorers introduced these hot peppers to Europe, Africa and Asia. These peoples used them and developed their own spicy dishes. They also developed medicinal uses as well as culinary uses for this herb.

Cayenne is hot and spicy and used a lot in cooking. The heat is caused by a substance called capsaicin. Capsaicin has been studied for its pain relieving properties, and its cardiovascular benefits. Cayenne is also very effective for opening up congested nasal cavities.

Cayenne has vitamin A in it and this includes beta-carotene which is helpful for asthma, osteoarthritis and rheumatoid arthritis. It also is an antioxidant which helps prevent free radicals which can lead to atherosclerosis, colon cancer, and diabetic problems like nerve damage and heart disease. Cayenne is rich in Vitamin C, and contains some minerals like iron, copper and potassium.

Cayenne has been used to fight inflammation. It inhibits a substance in the body called substance P, a substance that has been linked to the process that causes inflammation. Cayenne is being studied for treatment of pain associated with psoriasis, arthritis, and diabetic neuropathy. It also appears to help cluster headaches.

Cayenne has benefits for the cardiovascular system. They include lowering cholesterol, triglycerides, platelet aggregation and fibrin. Cultures where hot peppers like cayenne are used extensively have a lower rate of heart attack, stroke, and pulmonary embolism.

Cayenne can be good for heart health. Capsaicin, the active ingredient in cayenne, can thin the blood if it is taken on a regular basis. In an emergency it has the opposite effect and cayenne, when given during a heart attack can stop the clotting of the blood in the arteries

The capsaicin in peppers is great for clearing out the sinuses and very useful for coughs and colds. A tea made of hot cayenne pepper and garlic helps the sinuses drain and relieves congestion.

Cayenne has been used for losing weight. The heat generated by the consumption of the pepper produces the burning of calories. This is because thermogenesis is created, and oxygen consumption is increased for up to 20 minutes or more after it is taken.

Cayenne is good for arthritis. There are many cream and ointment formulations on the market with capsaicin as the main ingredient that can be put on the areas that are painful.

Cayenne is a useful herb/spice to have around in an emergency. It helps blood clot when a cut is bleeding. Put the cayenne right on the wound to stop the bleeding then cover the wound with a bandage.

Side Effects:

Cayenne is in the nightshade family, and if you have problems consuming nightshades then it is better to stay away from cayenne.

Be careful using cayenne topically unless it is in a lotion, cream or ointment. It can cause burning and itching of the skin. Don't use on the sensitive skin around the eyes and do not apply to damaged or broken skin.

Very little research has been done regarding oral use of cayenne for children. It is probably best not to give it to them. Consult your health care provider.

Stop cayenne 2 weeks before surgery. It may cause excessive bleeding. Always consult your health care practitioner.

Recipes

Cayenne Tea

½ to 1 t of cayenne pepper (depending on how strong you want it).

1 C water

Heat water to boiling. Pour over cayenne pepper in a cup

Drink slowly and let it slide down your throat.

Cayenne, Chicken and Garlic Broth (This is really good for clearing out your nasal passages if you have a cold or the flu.)

1 t cayenne pepper

1-2 t minced garlic

1-2 t chicken bullion

Cayenne and Green Bean Stir Fry

1 C fresh sliced tomatoes

½ t cayenne pepper (more if desired)

2 C green beans fresh or frozen.

Toss together in a wok or frying pan. Cook 7-10 minutes depending on how crunchy you like your beans.

Serve and enjoy!

Cayenne Weight Loss Drink

Cayenne pepper

Lemon juice

Sweetener of choice (stevia, agave, maple syrup, honey)

Mix in proportions as desired. Drink for weight loss.

Measure the ingredients into a large cup or a soup bowl with a handle on it. Pour boiling water over it and mix it up. Drink at your leisure.

Additional Uses:

Bleeding - Cayenne powder can be sprinkled on cuts and abrasions to stop the bleeding. It does not burn.

Discourage animals - Cayenne pepper can be useful to repel wildlife like squirrels, rabbits and deer.

Tea - Cayenne added to chicken soup will help clean out your sinuses. Cayenne can be made into a tea with horseradish for the same purpose.

4) Sage

Let's move now from South America to the Mediterranean. There are many herbs that come from this part of the world, such as lavender, rosemary, sweet basil and thyme. They all belong to the *Lamiaceae* family. The Latin name for sage is *Salvia Officinalis* which means "to save".

During the time of the bubonic plague in Europe, thieves developed a concoction containing sage that was called Four Thieves Vinegar which was said to prevent them from getting the plague. Sage was also used as a meat preservative before the days of refrigeration. It was thought that sage warded off evil spirits and the Emperor Charlemagne recommended it for cultivation. During the middle ages it was cultivated in monastery gardens and used for healing purposes.

According to folklore, sage is good for many things; nervous disorders, memory, digestive problems, mental disorders, Alzheimer's' Disease, and depression. In modern times research has been done regarding the use of sage for Alzheimer's and preliminary findings are promising. Sage is anti-inflammatory and may help Type 2 diabetes. It has also been widely used for relieving the hot flashes of menopause. Sage has properties that are tonic, astringent, diaphoretic, and stimulant.

Sage oil is good for stiff muscles, rheumatism and neuralgia. Sage is sometimes used topically for eczema and skin injuries. Sage is also anti-viral, anti-fungal, and antibacterial. Sage is used in aromatherapy to relieve headaches, stress, nervousness and anxiety. Sage can soothe indigestion and it can be made into an herbal tea that can serve as a good mouthwash. Rubbing sage leaves on your teeth can whiten them and combat bad breath. It is good for gum disease and throat infections.

Sage has been used as a hot decoction for colds and flu, and it can act as a diaphoretic. This is good because the sweating helps your body get rid of toxins. Sage has also been used as a cold infusion that can decrease sweating and it also can stop diarrhea.

Sage can dry up breast milk, so it is not recommended for a mother who is nursing, however it can be useful for a mother who is weaning an older baby. Sage can also be useful for hot flashes that come with menopause.

Sage comes in capsules, teas, oils, and tinctures. Sage tea can be blended with other herbs like lavender, mint, and catnip. This herb has many nutritional benefits. It contains folic acid, pyridoxine, vitamin A, vitamin C, vitamin k, zinc, iron, calcium, copper, manganese, magnesium, potassium, and flavonoids. It has antioxidant properties.

Side Effects:

The use of large quantities of sage can cause nervous irritation, convulsions, and death and should not be used by people with epileptic conditions. It should not be used in pregnancy because it stimulates the uterus and may cause miscarriage. Sage can cause irritation and dry mouth.

Sage has a constituent called thujone and if sage is taken for a long period of time it can cause confusion and an increase in heart rate. To avoid this only take sage under a health care professional's guidance for a short period of time like 1-2 weeks, then stop for awhile. Be sure and talk to your health care provider about whether or not using sage is right for you. Sage can increase blood pressure in some people. It can interact with diabetes medicines, and sedative medicines so proceed with caution and check it out with your health care provider.

Recipes

Sore Throat Gargle

1 T of dried sage leaves

1 pint boiling water

Bring to a boil and let it steep for about 15 minutes. Strain, and add honey or sweetener of choice. Use as a gargle two times a day.

Sage Tea

1 t dried sage

2 C boiling water

Lemon if desired

Add sage to boiling water. Remove from heat. Add honey, maple syrup or desired sweetener because sage alone tastes bitter.

NOTE: Sage can be mixed with black tea for flavor and variety. Also, you can combine it with rosemary or thyme or lavender and some lemon zest. Experiment with different ingredients and see what you like best. An infusion is more concentrated than a tea and you need to

33

add more sage and let it steep longer. Infusions are usually used for medicinal purposes.

Sage and Fennel Tea (good for sore throat, colds and flu)

1 oz. sage leaves

¾ oz. fennel seeds

1 C water, boiled

Make a mixture of the sage leaves and fennel seeds. Use 1 ½ t of the mixture and pour the boiling water over it. Let steep 2-3 minutes. Drink slowly and let it slide down your throat. A variation of this can be made using mint instead of fennel. Sweeteners and/or lemon can be added as desired

Additional uses:

After shave – Sage has astringent properties and can be used as an after shave.

Gargle – sage tea can be mixed with a small amount of cider vinegar and used as a gargle for sore throats, laryngitis and tonsillitis.

Gray hair - In the past sage was used to darken gray hair. It is good for your scalp and the hair feels soft and shiny.

Indigestion – sage tea can be used for digestion problems and flatulence.

5) Rosemary

Rosemary, *Rosmarinus officinalis,* is another herb from the Mediterranean area. It is in the mint family, *Lamiaceae*, and is an evergreen. Rosemary is used for flavoring food and beverages and it is used in cosmetics. It is a good herb for cooking meat, and seems to be especially good with lamb. Some recent research appears to suggest that it has anti-cancer properties. Rosemary is anti-bacterial, anti-inflammatory, anti-fungal, and antiseptic.

In past history rosemary was known as the "herb of remembrance". The ancients used it for strengthening the memory. The first we know of rosemary was around 5000 BCE. The Romans would put sprigs of rosemary on the graves of loved ones to show that they would be remembered. During the time of the Tudors in England, brides would wear rosemary to signify that they would not forget their families or the life they had before their marriage.

Pliny (23-79 AD), Dioscorides, and Galen famous healers in ancient times all wrote about rosemary. It was popular for flavoring meats during the Middle Ages. Rosemary was thought to protect folks against the bubonic plague of the 1600's, and was mentioned in the writings of both

Shakespeare and Sir Thomas Moore. There is an old saying about "Where rosemary flourishes the lady rules." However, husbands destroying the plant did not usually bring relief from their wives rule. Rosemary was burned during religious ceremonies and in the rooms of the sick to purify the air.

Rosemary is credited with helping memory and recall. Ophelia in Shakespeare's Hamlet speaks of rosemary being for remembrance. Scholars in ancient Greece would wear wreaths of rosemary to help them in their exams.

In modern times rosemary is recognized for its medicinal uses. It contains salicylic acid and is considered by many to be useful for arthritis. It is also used for skin problems, like dandruff. Rosemary is being researched for potential anti-cancer properties and may be useful for preventing and treating Alzheimer's disease.

Rosemary is said to stimulate the hair-follicles and help prevent premature balding but there is no research to back that up. However, research does show that it is good for dandruff. Rosemary is said to reverse graying hair. It stimulates the roots of the hair and increases blood flow to the head. This promotes growth and prevents breakage.

Rosemary tea is good for headaches, colds and depression. It is tonic, astringent, diaphoretic, and is a stimulant. The oil can be used externally for gout and rheumatism. It is good for anxiety and it is good for mild memory impairment.

Some of the nutritional benefits of rosemary include dietary fiber, Vitamins A, B-6, C, D, E and K, as well as pyridoxine, folic acid, pantothenic acid, and minerals like potassium, calcium, iron, manganese, and copper and magnesium. It is high in antioxidants. Rosemary contains a substance called rosmarinic acid which is anti-inflammatory. Rosemary also contains fiber.

Rosemary contains substances that stimulate the immune system and that help digestion. It can reduce the severity of asthma attacks, and it appears to increase blood flow to the brain, improving concentration. Another interesting property of rosemary is that it seems to make hair grow faster.

Rosemary is considered good for staving off the aging process because it is an ingredient in skin preparations and is known to rejuvenate the skin. It sharpens mental clarity and stimulates the function of the brain. For many people rosemary is good for long- term memory. It has been used by students to help them retain memory of their studies longer.

Rosemary cleanses the system by helping the liver to function better. Rosemary can calm down an upset stomach, and relieve muscle pain. It can help you fight stress and anxiety by helping you to relax. It can be applied topically for arthritis, sore muscles, and pain in the joints and muscles. It is good for indigestion, and helps prevent food borne illness if it is taken with meat or eggs. It is also a mild diuretic and helps kidney function.

Side Effects:

The use of Rosemary as a medicine for children does not have research to back it up, so do not give it to children under 18 years of age. It is safe for children to eat foods that have rosemary spice in them.

Do not take more than 6g of dried rosemary per day. Do not take rosemary oil because it is toxic. Caution is recommended for women who are pregnant, because rosemary can cause miscarriage. It is also not recommended for nursing mothers.

Do not take rosemary if you have high blood pressure, ulcerative colitis, or Chron's disease. Rosemary may interfere with blood thinners like Warfarin, ACE inhibitors for high blood pressure, and diabetes medicines. As always, check with your health care provider before using rosemary therapeutically.

Recipes:

Rosemary Tea

1 t rosemary

1 C boiling water

Steep 4-5 minutes or longer if you want it stronger. Drink and enjoy.

NOTE: You can combine the rosemary with lavender or thyme to make a tasty beverage. You can also add lemon and/or honey to make a good beverage.

Biscuits with Rosemary

2 C baking mix (Biscuit mix is good)

½ tsp sugar

¾ c milk

2 Tb Butter

2 t dried rosemary, crumbled up

Mix ingredients with baking mix. Add more or less milk as need to get soft dough. Roll out dough to 1/2 inch thickness on a lightly floured surface. Cut into biscuit rounds and put on a greased and floured baking sheet. Bake according to directions on the baking mix package.

Potatoes with Rosemary

1 lb. potatoes (Yukon Gold is good but you can use any kind.

2 T olive oil

1 t salt

5 t chopped fresh rosemary with stems removed (you can use dried rosemary but there is nothing like the taste of fresh)

½ t ground pepper (more or less as desired)

Chop the potatoes into small cubes and completely coat with the olive oil. Add rosemary, salt and pepper. Garlic may be added if desired. Stir well. Turn into a baking dish that has been sprayed with non-stick spray. Use a fairly large dish so potatoes are spread out instead of bunched on top of each other, (unless you want to stir them more often while they are baking). Bake 45 minutes stirring them once or twice until golden brown. Use the broiler towards the end if you like them crispy. Remove from oven and serve. This goes well with steak.

Additional uses:

Air freshener - Rosemary can be used for air freshener. You can make potpourri with rosemary.

Baldness - According to folklore, rosemary is a remedy for baldness, though there is no scientific evidence for this.

Bath - For a soothing bath for sore muscles you can take 2 cups of rosemary and make an infusion. Let it steep for 20 minutes and add to your bath. Epsom salts can also be added if desired.

Congestion – For congestion in the respiratory tract, breathe in the scent of rosemary oil. You can also boil rosemary in water, place it in a bowl, put a towel over your head and breathe in the steam. This is also good for stuffed up sinuses.

Dandruff - A strong infusion of Nettle leaf and rosemary can be used as an herbal rinse for hair and fights dandruff. It can speed hair growth and it conditions your scalp. Use it as a rinse after washing.

Diffuser - You can use rosemary essential in a diffuser. It is said to help folks maintain their focus, good in the workplace.

Eyes - Use wet rosemary tea bags for puffy eyes. Apply bags to eyelids for 10 minutes. Wash face afterwards to prevent skin staining.

Mouthwash - Rosemary can be used as a mouthwash. Steep rosemary in 2 c of water, Strain and use. It may be refrigerated.

6) Thyme

Thyme, *Thymus Vulgaris*, is another Mediterranean herb/spice that is very popular in cooking. It is a perennial plant that is used in Italian, Greek, Spanish and French cooking. There are several varieties of thyme. I like lemon thyme. Thyme has many medicinal uses such as treating infections and using thyme oil in cough syrups. It is antiseptic, antibacterial and antifungal.

Thyme is another spice that was used a lot by the Greeks and Romans. In Roman times thyme was used for the culture of bees. The Egyptians used it in embalming, to preserve the dead bodies of their pharaohs and other important people. They also used it in their baths. They used it for depression, and to lift the mood.

Thyme was considered by the Romans to be an antidote for poison. It was a favorite of the emperors for that reason and a bath in warm water with thyme was thought to stop the effects of poison if it was accidentally consumed.

In the Middle Ages thyme was grown in monastery gardens for use in cooking. Thyme was used to preserve meat before refrigeration and thyme oil was used to treat consumption. When the bubonic plague struck in the 14th century people used thyme for relief and prevention. The famous herbalist Culpeper suggested using thyme for nightmares. In Victorian times a patch of thyme was a place where fairies had danced during the night.

Thyme can help digestive problems and prevent flatulence. It is antispasmodic and relieves menstrual cramping. Tea made of thyme can help a hangover, and it is often used for sore throats, colds, and reducing respiratory inflammation. It has been used to clear congestion.

Thyme is good for relieving bronchitis. It has been used as a base for formulating a mouthwash that is used in treating dental cavities and gingivitis. Thyme contains antioxidants, one of which is lutein, which is good for your eyes. It also contains B-complex vitamins, vitamins A, K, E, and C and folic acid, as well as calcium, potassium, manganese, magnesium, iron, and selenium.

Thyme can be used for pink eye or conjunctivitis. It works to eliminate lice and can help with gastroenteritis. Thyme is good for fatigue, and stress. Thyme contains antioxidants and flavonoids that neutralize free radicals in the body. Thyme is useful for Alzheimer's disease, arthritis, and is an anti-fungal that is good for athlete's foot. Thyme tea is good for emphysema, asthma, and hay fever.

Thyme is good for digestion and combats parasites such as hookworms and tapeworms. Thyme is good for reducing the pain of arthritis. Hot thyme tea can be used to induce menstruation. For this reason it should not be used during pregnancy.

Thyme is a diaphoretic which means it induces perspiration, and as a febrifuge which means it can bring down a fever.

I could go on and on, but I think you get the picture. Thyme is a mighty good herb and is good for a lot of things, even hand sanitizer and acne treatment.

Side Effects:

If you have Allergic Reactions to plants in the *Lamiaceae* family, avoid drinking tea made from thyme. Some of the side effects of large doses of thyme include heartburn, nausea, diarrhea, upset stomach, headache and dizziness.

Folks are cautioned to be careful about drinking thyme tea if they have a history of heart disease, peptic ulcers and gastrointestinal problems. The amounts used in cooking are usually considered to be safe.

There has not been a lot of research on the effects of thyme on pregnant women or nursing mothers. If you are pregnant consult your health care provider before using thyme tea or supplements.

Recipes

Thyme Tea Recipe

1 tsp of dried thyme leaves, or 2 tsp fresh thyme leaves

2 cups of boiled fresh water.

Let steep 4-5 minutes.

Sweeten to taste with honey, or stevia, or agave syrup.

For variation use lemon thyme, or add lemon to regular thyme.

Rice with Lemon Thyme

1 T butter

1 C rice, I prefer brown rice

1 can organic, chicken broth

1 T lemon juice

1 T Thyme, fresh is preferred

Melt butter and stir in rice. Cook rice, until browned about 5 minutes. Mix chicken broth, lemon juice and thyme into rice. Cover and reduce heat to low. Cook until liquid has been absorbed. Fluff and serve. For variations add chopped onion, or olives, or shredded chicken, or parmesan cheese.

Rice with Chicken and Thyme

2 C cooked rice (I use brown rice, but you can use white)

1 or 2 C of fresh mushrooms (depending on how well you like mushrooms)

3 t olive oil

1 onion diced

2 t ground thyme

½ t poultry seasoning

Salt and pepper to taste

1 1/2 C diced chicken cooked

½ C chicken stock

½ C sour cream

1/2 C grated parmesan

2 C cheese (A Mexican blend is good, also cheddar works)

Cook the rice and preheat oven to 375 degrees

48

Slice mushrooms and put them in a pan with 2 t of the olive oil and sauté. Add mushrooms and continue to sauté. Add thyme, poultry seasoning, salt, and pepper. Let flavors mix and cook for a minute or so. Dice chicken. In a bowl mix the sauté mix and chicken. Add the rice. Mix. In a separate bowl mix together the sour cream, chicken stock and parmesan cheese and 1 c of the grated cheese. Stir this mixture into the mushroom and rice mixture. Use the remaining olive oil to oil a 2 qt. casserole dish. Put mixture into casserole dish. Bake 25 minutes. Sprinkle the rest of the cheese on top of the casserole and bake until cheese starts to brown. Remove from oven and serve hot.

Additional Uses:

Antiseptic - Fresh thyme leaves can be crushed and applied to cuts and wounds. It is a natural antiseptic.

Bath - Thyme can be added to a hot bath to relieve pain of body aches.

Colds and bronchitis - Thyme can be added to hot water when it is steaming. Inhaling the steam can help folks suffering from colds and bronchitis. It clears the respiratory airways.

Cosmetic - Thyme has a lot of hygienic and cosmetic uses. It is added to shampoos, and soaps.

Cuts and wounds - Strong thyme tea can be used as an antiseptic on external cuts and wounds.

Digestion remedy - Mix equal amounts of thyme, red clover, sage and rosemary. If you have nausea, add some sliced ginger.

Fungus - A tea made from thyme can be externally applied with a cotton ball to athletes' foot and toenail fungus.

Gum disease - Thyme tea is a good gargle or rinse for gum disease.

Infected eyes - Thyme tea bags can be used like a compress on infected eyes.

7) Basil

Basil *Ocimum basilicum* is also known as sweet basil. This is different from holy basil, *Basilicum sanctum*, which is used extensively in India and is a related species. Basil and its variations are thought to have originated in India. Basil is used extensively in Ayurvedic medicine, the ancient medicine of India. It was also used in Chinese medicine to promote blood circulation after birth, kidney problems and stomach cramps. A variety of basil called Holy Basil is considered sacred in India.

In Greek lore basil represents hatred and in European lore it is sometimes called the symbol of Satan. The famous herbalist Culpeper cites "Hilarius" a French physician as saying basil breeds scorpions in the brain. Basil is placed in the hands of the dead in Europe and in India it is placed in the mouth of the dying to make sure they reach God. The ancient Egyptians thought it would open the gates of heaven for a person who had died.

Basil has been used to help bronchitis, osteoarthritis, anxiety, insomnia, stress, indigestion and general pain. Basil helps lower blood pressure, ease tension and stress, relieve spasms, act as a detoxification agent, and as a cleanser for the blood. It is said to lower blood sugar. Basil may ease anxiety, work as an anti-inflammatory, lower cholesterol, and as an adaptogen, which means it can help the body adapt and bounce back.

According to folk lore the benefits of basil include: stimulating the brain, clearing the mind, aiding concentration, increasing endurance and stamina, resisting infection, improving blood circulation, and increasing the production of breast milk. Basil has a mild soothing effect that helps with nervousness and irritability, anxiety, depression and insomnia.

Basil can ease constipation, stomach cramps, indigestion, vomiting, and nausea from chemotherapy. It can help whooping cough, hiccups, headaches and migraines, depression, fevers, colds, influenza, coughs and sinusitis. It can also ease cramps in the uterus and intestines, aid with insomnia and it has been used to treat epilepsy; though I wouldn't recommend it for epilepsy without consulting a physician first.

Basil is good for gastrointestinal problems, like flatulence, cramping, colic, nausea and vomiting, worms, and parasites. Basil can be used to treat migraine, whooping cough, skin disorders, and as an insect repellent, as well as for insect bites. Basil is sometimes used for arthritis and rheumatism. It is antibacterial, and antiseptic.

There are a number of cultures where basil is used to promote menstruation, and induce labor. Some think it is an aphrodisiac; however there is no scientific evidence for this. Basil is anti-inflammatory and brings relief to things like aches and pains and inflamed bowels.

Basil contains a lot of nutrients. Among them are Vitamins A, C, K, iron, calcium, fiber, manganese, copper, magnesium, flavonoids and volatile oils. Basil is anti-bacterial and the essential oil will slow the growth of bad bacteria like staphylococcus that have become resistant to antibiotics. It also contains protein, and fiber.

Basil is a carminative which means it is good for flatulence; it is good for fevers, and for catarrh. It helps genito-urinary disorders and helps to relieve constipation. Basil oil works against mosquitoes and flies. It has been used as an antidote for poison, for French liquors, perfumes, and as a gourmet seasoning.

Side Effects:

Sweet basil has been known to enhance the effect of insulin and medicines that lower blood glucose. People with diabetes should be cautious with basil and consult with their health care provider.

Pregnant and nursing women should not use basil in larger amounts than that found in food. Always consult your health care practitioner.

Recipes:

Basil Tea

1 c boiling water

1 t dried basil or 2 t fresh

Pour boiling water over basil leaves and steep for 5 minutes. You can steep for a longer or shorter period of time depending on how strong you want it. For variation you can add lemon or lemon peel as desired. Strain, drink and enjoy.

For an infusion, steep for 15 minutes. Do not have more than 2 cups of the infusion a day and do not take it for more than ten days without a break for several days.

Tomato Rice Basil soup

1 can diced tomatoes

2/3 C cooked rice (I prefer brown but white is ok)

4 C tomato juice

12 leaves of fresh basil

1 C whipping cream

½ C olive oil (or butter if you prefer

Salt and pepper to taste

Puree tomatoes, basil and tomato juice and simmer for 30 minutes. Stir in heavy cream and butter or olive oil. Season as desired. Let soup simmer for 5-10 minutes, serve.

Additional uses:

Asthma and bronchitis - The essential oil can also be used as a chest rub.

Bath - Five or ten drops of basil essential oil can be added to bath water for relaxation.

Cold and bronchitis - The decoction of basil mixed with honey and ginger is an effective remedy for asthma, influenza, cough, cold and bronchitis

Foot bath - Pour boiling water over basil leaves for a pain-relieving foot-bath.

Headache - Rub crushed basil leaves into your temples to relieve headaches.

Insect bites - Crushed leaves can be used fresh for insect bites by rubbing the leaves on the bites to reduce inflammation and itching.

Insect repellent - The essential oil of basil can be applied externally as an insect repellent.

Inhalation - For head colds, the steam of basil leaves that have been in boiling water can be inhaled.

Warts - Basil leaves have traditionally been used to remove warts.

8) Oregano

Yet another herb from the Mediterranean area of the world, oregano, is known as *Oreganum vulgare* in Latin. It also comes from the *Lamiacea* family, which is also known as the mint family. The mint family is a large family of plants that includes sage, rosemary, thyme, marjoram and lemon balm.

The Greeks believed Aphrodite invented oregano to make man's life happier. They also put it on graves to give the departed spirits peace. Hippocrates used Oregano for stomach and respiratory disorders. The Romans adopted it from the Greeks and it spread to Europe and North Africa. It was used to spice meat and fish and it was used as a flavoring for wine.

Oregano was used in China as a medicinal herb for fever, vomiting, diarrhea, and itchy skin. In the United States, oregano was not common until after WW II when the soldiers came back from the war. It was mostly associated with pizza.

Oregano is antibacterial, antibiotic, antiviral and antifungal. The oregano oil is an especially strong antibacterial, and it is an antioxidant. It contains Vitamins C, E, and K as well as copper magnesium, calcium, and several of the B vitamins, iron and potassium, and Vitamin A.

Oregano stimulates bile flow and relieves flatulence. It is antiseptic and often used for coughs, tonsillitis, bronchitis and asthma. It is used by herbalists for women's problems and can be applied topically to toothache and aching joints.

Oregano has been used as a disinfectant and for itching skin. Oregano oil is very potent and is also anti-microbial. It helps kill intestinal parasites. It has been used for fungal infections like Candida. It has also been used for diarrhea, nausea, and jaundice and vomiting.

Oregano can be used to get rid of head lice. Oregano is an antioxidant which helps to slow down age related problems like nervousness, and degeneration of the muscles. According to researchers, a tablespoon of fresh oregano contains as much antioxidant as a medium sized apple. It is said to be used for such diseases of aging, heart disease, high blood pressure, macular degeneration and geriatric muscle deterioration.

Oregano has been used for colds, as a decongestant, for a sore throat, and for infected sinuses. It acts as an anti-inflammatory and can be used for cough. Oregano is often used for digestive complaints, such as an upset stomach, and diarrhea. It can kill parasites. Oregano is good for relieving minor aches and pains. It is good for skin problems like fungal infections and nail fungus. Oregano oil is used for menstrual problems in women. Oregano is known for strengthening the immune system.

Oregano has culinary uses and is used in many Italian dishes for seasoning. It is a standard spice for pizza.

Side Effects:

Do not use on sensitive or broken skin. If Oregano is taken in doses that are too high it can cause hives and itching.

Oregano for medicinal purposes is not recommended for pregnant or nursing women or for children. Always seek guidance from your health care practitioner.

If oil of oregano is used for a long time it may interfere with the absorption of iron by the body. Take the dosage recommended by your health care provider.

Be careful using oregano for children. Start with small doses. Be sure to discuss it with your doctor before starting use.

Recipes

Oregano Tea

1 1/2 t dried oregano leaves, or 2 ½ t fresh leaves

8 oz. boiling water

1 t honey (or sweetener of choice).

Place oregano leaves in boiling water and steep for 5 minutes. Steeping it longer will cause the tea to be bitter.

Strain into a mug. Add sweetener to taste. Stir and drink.

Oregano tea is good for sore throats and colds.

Variation for sinus congestion, skip the honey and add a drop or two of lime juice.

Meatball Soup with Fresh Oregano

5 cups vegetable broth

2 carrots diced

2 stalks celery diced

1 ½ t cumin

2 T chopped oregano

¼ t salt'

¼ t pepper

Turkey Meatballs (you can get prepared meatballs at the market or you can make your own)

Heat broth, carrots and celery in a covered pot until it comes to a boil. Add meatballs to soup. Reduce heat to a simmer and cook till carrots are tender. Stir in fresh oregano. Oregano is best fresh, though dried can be used. For a variation add a half cup brown rice if desired.

Additional Uses:

Add to meat – Adding oregano to meat before cooking can reduce toxic compounds.

Athletes foot – Massage oregano oil into feet. Add a drop or two to your socks and shoes.

Gargle - Oregano can be used as a gargle for a sore tooth or a sore throat.

Hand wash - Add a few drops to liquid soaps for washing your hands to fight germs and bacteria on your hands.

Head Lice – Add a couple drops of oregano oil to shampoo to wash head and scalp.

Mouthwash - A useful mouthwash can be made by adding a few drops to water and swishing through the mouth. It will destroy bad bacteria that grow in the mouth and help prevent tooth decay.

Sinus infection - For a sinus infection, inhale steam from a bowl of hot water with a few drops of oregano oil in it.

Sinusitis - For sinusitis or sore throat you can use a medicine dropper and put 2-3 drops under your tongue.

Sore throat - For a sore throat put 2-3 drops of oregano oil in orange juice

9) Turmeric

The Latin name for turmeric is *Curcuma Longa.* It is a member of the ginger family *Zingiberaceae.* It comes from Asia and is used a lot in India. It is a bright yellow color and is used for curries, rice, and chutneys, and it is also used as a dye for cloth. Turmeric gives mustard its yellow color and has lots of medicinal uses. It was called Indian saffron because its deep yellow color is similar to that of saffron.

Turmeric originated in Indonesia and Southern India and has been used for thousands of years. It was a very highly regarded herb in Ayurvedic medicine, the ancient medicine of India. Arab traders brought it to Europe in the 13th century. In Traditional Chinese medicine it was used for depression. In the western world it was not very popular until modern times; especially when studies showed it may help Alzheimer's disease as well as a number of other conditions.

Curcumin is the main constituent of turmeric and it contains anti-inflammatory, antiseptic, antibacterial, and antioxidant properties. It is thought to be useful for Alzheimer's disease because of its' extensive use in India where there is a very low incidence of this disease. Turmeric has the potential to help arthritis, and colitis, and neutralize toxins in smoke.

Turmeric is very good for detoxifying the liver. Turmeric is a natural pain killer and it may help psoriasis and other skin diseases. Turmeric can be used for heartburn, diarrhea, stomach bloating, headaches, bronchitis, colds, lung infections, fibromyalgia, leprosy, fever and menstrual problems. It also can be used for water retention, worms, kidney problems, flatulence, jaundice, and hemorrhage

Turmeric is very nutritious containing vitamins C, E, and K as well as minerals such as sodium, calcium, copper potassium, iron, magnesium and zinc.

Curcumin is a powerful antioxidant and can neutralize free radicals which can cause damage in the body. It is a useful herb that helps many chronic diseases like arthritis, heart disease, and stroke. Epidemiological studies suggest that the frequent use of turmeric can lower the incidence of breast, prostate, lung, and colon cancer. Turmeric is thought to support the liver.

There appears to be growing evidence that suggests that turmeric may be useful for Alzheimer's disease. In India the incidence of this disease is very low. In studies with mice turmeric appears to slow progression of this disease by slowing or preventing the formation of the amyloid-B plaques in the brain that are characteristic of Alzheimer's disease.

Side Effects:

People who have gallstones or bile obstruction should not take turmeric. Also, pregnant women should consult their doctor before taking turmeric in medicinal doses. Turmeric may exacerbate problems with stomach ulcers. People should always consult their health care provider, especially if they have serious heart and liver problems.

Turmeric can cause nausea and diarrhea with long term use. Turmeric may interfere with some medicines like aspirin, NSAID's, statins, diabetes drugs, blood pressure drugs and blood thinners. Don't give turmeric to children unless a doctor ok's it.

Recipes:

Turmeric Tea

1 c water

1 t turmeric

lemon and/or honey to taste

Boil water. Add turmeric and simmer for 10 minutes. Strain into a mug with cheesecloth and add honey and/or lemon to taste.

This tea is good if you feel you are catching a cold or the flu. It also lessens inflammation.

Longevity Tea

1 t turmeric powder

4 C water

Boil water and add turmeric. Let it simmer for 10 minutes, strain, and add ginger and/or honey to taste.

Turmeric Milk (good for relaxation)

1 C coconut milk

½ t ground turmeric

2 t sweetener of choice (honey, agave, maple syrup, stevia)

½ cinnamon stick, or ground cinnamon

Pinch black pepper

Put turmeric and milk in a saucepan and bring to a boil. Stir to combine. Reduce heat and simmer 20-30 minutes. Strain if necessary. Add sweetener and cinnamon. Add a pinch of black pepper and/or vanilla if desired. Serves 1

Additional Uses:

Cold or flu – Mix 1 t of turmeric powder in a glass of milk and drink.

Cuts and burns – Turmeric powder sprinkled on a cut or burn can speed up the healing process.

Curry powder – Blend your own secret recipe.

Dye Easter eggs – Turmeric is a dye and can be used for numerous things.

Face mask – Mix some turmeric with yogurt and honey. Apply to the skin for 20 minutes.

Homemade soap – Turmeric can add color to the soap and it is good for your skin.

Scrambled eggs or tofu – Add a pinch of turmeric to add to the flavor.

Sunburn - A paste made of turmeric can be applied to sunburn. It is also used in sunscreens.

10) Clove

Clove, which in the Latin classification is called, *Syzugium aromaticum,* is a member of the *Myrtacea* family. Clove trees originated in the Spice Islands and now cloves are grown all over the world.

The clove comes from the dried flower bud of the clove tree. Cloves are used extensively in cooking and are also used for medicinal remedies. The name clove came from the French word *clov*, which means nail. This is because a clove resembles a nail.

Archeologists have found cloves in a ceramic vessel in Syria, dating back to approximately the 3rd century BCE. In 200 BCE cloves came to China from Java. The emperor required that his visitors take a clove and hold it in their mouth to freshen their breath before an audience with him. The Romans used cloves for fragrance and perfume.

In the middle ages Europeans used cloves to preserve and flavor food. In the 16th century Magellan sailed around the world and claimed the Spice Islands for Portugal. In the 17th century the Dutch took over the clove business from the Portuguese and destroyed all clove trees except for those on two islands. This was to help them maintain their monopoly in the clove trade. In the second half of the 18th century the French smuggled cloves from the East Indies and took them to the new world, breaking the Dutch monopoly. Cloves are mentioned in the *Arabian Nights* and the Muslims traded with India for cloves.

Cloves used for medicinal purposes are perhaps best known for relieving the pain of a toothache if you are unable to get to a dentist right away. Cloves have been used for acne, and other skin conditions. Cloves are thought to relax the muscle lining of the stomach thereby bringing relief for digestive problems such as acid reflux.

Clove tea is used for bloating and gas as well as nausea and diarrhea. Cloves are used for toenail fungus and are also good for inflammation of the mouth and throat. The oils, flower buds, leaves and stems are used to make medicine. Cloves are anti-fungal, antiseptic, antiviral, anesthetic and are considered to be an aphrodisiac. Cloves are used for coughs, asthma and headaches.

Cloves are diaphoretic and can help relieve colds by causing perspiration for folks with fevers, sore throats and flu. They have also been taken for whooping cough. Cloves are good for mouth ulcers and sore gums. A gargle can be used for a sore throat. Cloves can relieve nausea and vomiting as well as flatulence. Clove oil can be applied to the skin for cuts and scrapes.

Side Effects:

Cloves are generally regarded as safe. Children should not take clove oil as it can cause serious health problems such as seizures and liver damage. Clove oil is safe when applied to the skin and mouth sparingly. Inhaling the smoke from clove cigarettes is not safe and can cause breathing problems and lung infections.

Dried clove can cause irritation of the mouth and damage to the dental tissues and it is unsafe to inject clove oil into the veins. Pregnant and nursing women can take cloves in normal amounts in food but should not use it as a medicine. Always consult your physician before using cloves as a medicine.

Clove seems to slow the clotting of the blood so it should not be taken if you are on blood thinners, or for 2 weeks before surgery. Some people are allergic to cloves. Again, talk it over with your doctor. Be careful about giving small children a clove to suck on. It can be a choking hazard.

Recipes:

Clove Tea

1 t crushed clove in a tea bag or infuser

1 C of boiling water

To prepare a clove tea, take a tea bag or infuser and fill it with crushed clove. Let it steep covered in a cup of water for 8 to 10 minutes. Milk and sweetener can be added as desired. Cloves are often used in Chai teas.

Clove Tea for Respiratory Congestion

2 cloves

1 stick cinnamon

Crushed cardamom seeds (1 or 2 seeds will do)

1 black tea bag

1 to 2 C water (depending on the size of your mug)

Place cloves, cinnamon and cardamom in an infuser. Place in mug with boiling water and steep 1 minute (steep longer for a stronger brew.)

Pumpkin Cookies with Clove, Cinnamon and Nutmeg

1 C pumpkin

½ C white sugar

½ C brown sugar

1 egg

2 C flour

2 t baking powder

2 t cinnamon

¼ t clove

¼ t nutmeg

½ t salt

½ t baking soda

1 t milk

1 t vanilla

2 C semi-sweet chocolate chips

½ c walnuts (if desired)

Combine pumpkin, sugar, oil and egg. Mix well. In a separate bowl add flour, baking powder, spices, salt, and baking soda. Combine the two mixtures. Add vanilla, chocolate chips and nuts. Drop on a greased cookie sheet and bake at 350 degrees for 10 to 12 minutes or until golden brown and firm.

Additional Uses:

Acne - For acne make a paste of clove powder and honey and apply to the affected area.

Bad Breath - Chewing on cloves can relieve bad breath

Cough - Chewing a clove with salt can relieve coughing.

Earache - For an earache mix clove oil and sesame oil. Warm the mixture and put 2-3 drops in the ear.

Indigestion - Drinking clove tea after a meal can ease indigestion.

Insect repellent - Clove oil diluted in a solution of water makes a good insect repellent.

Nausea – A cup of clove tea can relieve nausea and digestive problems.

Stomach ache - Clove oil taken with sugar is good for a stomach ache.

Throat congestion - Chewing a roasted clove is good for throat congestion. It is good for inflammation of the pharynx.

Toenail fungus – Apply clove oil directly to the skin or nails. The clove oil can be diluted with olive oil if you have sensitive skin.

Toothache - Press a clove between the jaws at the site of the toothache to ease pain.

Warts – Put a couple of drops of clove on a cotton ball or band-aid and place over a wart. Change it every day. After 3-4 weeks the wart should disappear.

For Further Reading

Aggarwal, Bharat, B., *Healing Spices How to use 50 Everyday Spices to Boost Health and Beat Disease,* 2011

David, Elizabeth, *Spices, Salt and Aromatics in the English Kitchen,* Penguin Books, New York, 1976

Dalby, Andrew, *Dangerous Tastes; the Story of Spices,* University of California Press, Berkeley, 2000

Hemphill, Ian, *Spice and Herb Bible, 3rd edition*, Robert Rose Publisher, Toronto Ontario Canada, 2014

Keay, John, *The Spice Route; A History*, University of California Press, Berkeley, 2006

Little, Brenda, *The Complete Book of Herbs & Spices,* Silverleaf Press, Utah, 2006

Simonds, Nina, *Spices of Life: Simple and delicious recipes for great health,* Alfred A. Knopf, New York, 2005

Stanway, Penny, *The Miracle of Spices, Practical Tips for Health and Home,* Watkins Publishing, London, 2013

Turner, Jack, *The History of a Temptation: Spice,* Vintage Books, New York, 2004

Send me an e-mail with your comments and check out my website and blog.

E-mail: valerielull923@gmail.com

Check out my website, www.valerielull.com

Check out my blog, www.vallull@blogspot.com

For a discount on my other book *Ten Healthy Teas* go to www.outskirtspress.com/bookstore

Also available at www.Amazon.com

If you enjoyed this book, write a review on Amazon and/or Goodreads.